When Nothing Else Works

How To Cure Your Lower Back Pain Fast!

When Nothing Else Works

How To Cure
Your Lower Back Pain Fast!

S. F. Howe

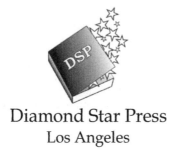

Diamond Star Press
Los Angeles

When Nothing Else Works: How To Cure Your Lower Back Pain Fast!

Second Edition – Paperback
Copyright © 2018 S. F. Howe

Published by Diamond Star Press
ISBN-13: 978-0-9774335-9-9
ISBN-10: 0-9774335-9-5

First Edition Copyright © 2011 S. F. Howe
First digital edition was authored by S. F. Howe writing as Kent Ellis and was titled, "Lower Back Pain Relief: The Amazing Story Of How I Cured My Chronic Lower Back Pain In Only Ten Days!

Books by S. F. Howe

Matrix Man
How To Become Enlightened, Happy And Free In An
Illusion World

The Bringer Discourses
On Waking Up to the Mind Control Programs of the
Matrix Reality

The Top Ten Myths Of Enlightenment
Exposing The Truth About Spiritual Enlightenment
That Will Set You Free!

Secrets Of The Plant Whisperer
How To Care For, Connect, And Communicate With
Your House Plants

Vision Board Success
How To Get Everything You Want With Vision
Boards!

Sex Yoga
The 7 Easy Steps To A Mind-Blowing Kundalini
Awakening!

Morning Routine For Night Owls
How To Supercharge Your Day With A Gentle Yet
Powerful Morning Routine!

Transgender America
Spirit, Identity, & The Emergence Of The Third
Gender

When Nothing Else Works
How To Cure Your Lower Back Pain Fast!

Free Gift

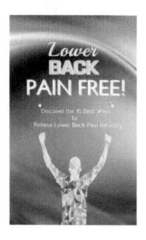

As my thanks to you for reading *When Nothing Else Works: How To Cure Your Lower Back Pain Fast!*, I would like you to have the special gift of a bonus ebook.

Your free gift, *Lower Back Pain Free!: Discover The 10 Best Ways to Cure Lower Back Pain Naturally*, is a compendium of natural cures that will offer you additional healing options to help free you from lower back pain. It's the perfect complement to *When Nothing Else Works.* Together, these two books will give you all the information you will ever need to maintain a healthy lower back.

To get your bonus ebook, just send an email to info@diamondstarpress.com with proof of purchase and "Send Lower Back Pain Gift" in the subject field, and we'll get your free gift out to you right away. Do it now before you forget!

For those who suffer from lower back pain and have long been searching for a natural solution

Table of Contents

Introduction

My Lower Back Pain Solution

You may be wondering what qualifies me to write a book on lower back pain. After all, I'm not a physician, a chiropractor, a nurse or a physical therapist. And you would be right to ask that question. So here is my answer: what qualifies me is that ten years ago I accidentally discovered a completely overlooked natural method of healing lower back pain. When I applied this quick and easy method to my own lower back pain in an attitude of experimentation, I found that after ten or eleven days, I was completely free of the severe, chronic pain that dogged me for an entire year. And better yet, the pain has not returned. Throughout the past ten years, I have been completely well and have had no complaints with my lower back.

When I realized how many people are living with terrible lower back pain or, in desperation, going under the knife to cure their lower back pain, not to mention taking side effects-laden medication prescribed by their doctor, I felt obliged to share my story. If this guide helps even one person to overcome their lower back pain, I will feel that this book has served its purpose.

My unique discovery is an idea so simple, so natural and so basic, it is completely overlooked. My technique requires no medication, no surgery, no equipment, no special environment, no doctor or therapist, no costs of any kind, and takes almost no time. Yet in a matter of days, it healed me completely after suffering for an entire year with debilitating, constant lower back pain.

In this book, you will get the complete lowdown on what I did to create a rapid healing of my own lower back pain. If you think this is going to be a difficult or time-consuming task, you're wrong! To accomplish the healing of my lower back pain, it involved using a dead simple method for only thirty seconds per day to start, then gradually increasing to five minutes per day over the next ten or eleven days. That was it. And to my astonishment, my lower back pain was gone, never to return.

May you find your lower back pain solution in the pages of this book. If you keep an open mind, you are likely to discover here the relief from suffering you may have been searching for, for a very long time. All I can say is, it worked for me and for many of my readers, and I believe it will work for you too!

I hope you enjoy learning about my lower back pain solution.

To your health!

Chapter 1

The Simple Lower Back Pain Cure They Don't Want You To Know About

I promised I would share with you how I cured my lower back pain quickly and easily. It all began in Monterey, California, approximately fen years ago. I was relaxing on a weekend holiday in that lovely seaside town. One thing I've noticed is that good ideas often pop into my mind when I've taken a break from the demands of my everyday life.

That Sunday morning on the last day of my vacation was no different. I woke up with thoughts about how infants develop not only their physiology but also their brains through crawling. As a psychologist, I knew from my studies in developmental psychology that crawling is critical to human development. It stimulates proper spinal development while integrating the left and right sides of the brain. This helps build the neural connections that eventually enable an infant to walk.

I also knew that crawling, a horizontal exercise, diminishes or even eliminates the negative effects of gravity on the human body. According to the scientific research, reptiles and mammals that crawl on four legs rarely exhibit cardiovascular, cerebrovascular or spinal diseases. I wondered whether crawling could also provide unique benefits for people with severe, chronic lower back pain.

Yes, I had been suffering severe lower back pain for over a year. I could find no specific cause nor was I able to find a cure. My weight was normal, I drank plenty of water, meditated for stress, took a variety of health supplements, ate a healthy diet and exercised daily. Even so, I was in constant pain. But being stubborn and averse to medical diagnoses and treatments, I had avoided going to the doctor. I feared being given strong painkillers and told I would need surgery. Instead, I was secretly praying for a solution.

When I was in pain, thinking about crawling was nothing new, as I would often get the urge to hit the floor on all fours. I resisted doing so, of course, because it felt unseemly, if not crazy. But that morning, logical or illogical as it may have been, I decided to give in to the urge to crawl. Because it didn't feel hygienic to do it on the hotel room floor, I threw the bedclothes off the firm king-size bed and began to crawl around the bed as best I could.

After I had done that for a few minutes, feeling utterly ridiculous, I stood up and to my surprise noticed that my spine seemed a bit straighter and stronger. I still had pain in my lower back, but overall it seemed slightly improved. I determined right then and there to try crawling on the floor when I got home.

Chapter 2

The Research Says It All

Thus began my fascination with crawling. Once home, I researched crawling on the Internet and found, to my amazement, that crawling had more health benefits than I ever imagined possible. The research showed that crawling was nothing less than a miracle cure for innumerable physical and neurological ailments, but that it was virtually ignored by the contemporary medical and fitness communities, having fallen to the wayside more than 60 years ago with the advent of new medications, new surgery techniques and new fitness trends. Obviously, new doesn't always mean better.

Here's what I learned about crawling: It's a single, very simple physical exercise that speeds up the metabolism, burns fat, causes weight loss, tones and strengthens the entire body, improves posture, strengthens the back, strengthens the core, tones abs, tones and strengthens the upper body, tones thighs and butt, gives an excellent cardio workout, improves lung function, relieves or eliminates aches and pains and improves the flexibility and function of joints. It is great for the sedentary and great for the active too.

But not only does it do all that, it also stimulates brain activity, facilitates right/left brain integration, improves mood, relieves depression, increases intelligence, memory, problem-solving and creativity, heals ADD and dyslexia, and has been used in the treatment of Parkinson's, stroke, mental retardation and brain injuries. In other words, it is the perfect anti-ageing exercise! Yet it can also be used effectively by virtually everyone, including kids.

To this day, army commandos are still being taught to bear crawl, which is a variation of crawling, as part of their basic conditioning. Crawling is still being used as therapy for victims of Parkinson's disease and cerebral palsy. And finally, it is still a popular treatment for children with attention deficit disorders.

The crawling champ of the universe, who competes against himself in an annual crawling competition in Italy, is the world's biggest proponent of crawling. He claims that its vast and far-reaching health benefits exceed any other remedy known to man, that its multitude of benefits have barely been explored, yet it will always be ignored by the mainstream solely because, to the human ego, it is an unattractive exercise.

But what does this have to do with your lower back pain, you ask? Everything, so stay with me. I just instinctively knew that the agility, power, strength and brain integration that crawling provided for army commandos, for those suffering from severe neuromuscular diseases and for children with neurological disorders, would help to heal my lower back. Armed with this information, I launched a daily program of crawling.

This is one of those instances where following my intuition – some call it listening to your inner voice, having a hunch or a feeling in your gut – led to a genuine breakthrough. For those who doubt the value of intuition, be sure to read Chapter Four: The Science Behind the Method. You will be pleased to know that my discovery is backed up by extensive scientific data, and you can learn more about the science by visiting the online sources cited at the end of that chapter and in the Resources section.

Chapter 3

My Daily Program

Based on my research, I knew I should crawl for no more than 30 seconds the first time. So I set the timer, determined my trajectory – up and down the living room on the living room carpet -- reminded myself to not lift my neck as it can cause a strain, and began.

I discovered that crawling was a demanding exercise at first, yet something we all instinctively know how to do. The type of crawling I did was the most fundamental -- on hands and knees, moving the right arm and left knee forward, followed by the left arm and right knee forward. This alternating sequence constitutes the basic crawling formula and can be performed as slowly as is necessary while you are building up your muscles and familiarity with the exercise.

After the very first crawling session, I could feel myself standing straighter, my spine more aligned. On day two, I may have crawled ten or twenty seconds longer than 30, and again felt that my spine was stronger and healthier. By day three, I set the timer for one minute and went back and forth in the living room on my hands and knees until the timer rang. At that point, I noticed that my knees felt sore during crawling and I determined to purchase a pair of knee pads to lessen the pressure of the floor against my knees.

On day four, I went to a Big Five sports store and purchased several different types of knee pads and knee protection devices. However, when I used them for crawling, I realized that none of them allowed a smooth or comfortable crawling experience and were not the right choice. I decided to visit Home Depot, where I looked for foam knee pads that workers use when doing jobs on their knees. I soon found and purchased inexpensive knee pads with Velcro attachments that could easily wrap around bare knees or around pants, which seemed like the ideal choice. In the resources section of this book, you will find information about obtaining knee pads.

By day five, I was crawling approximately two minutes and experimenting with speeding up and slowing down. The knee pads worked perfectly, completely eliminating any discomfort from contact with the floor. As always, my back felt straighter and stronger after the exercise and by now my lower back pain seemed to be diminishing.

I continued crawling daily for a total of ten or eleven days, never straining or forcing myself to do more than was comfortable, yet increasing the length of time of my crawling by 30 second increments when possible. I also experimented with a second crawling technique that uses a right arm with right knee movement followed by a left arm and left knee movement. Finally, I tried backwards crawling, using both types of arm and leg movements. But I never crawled for more than five minutes at a time.

By day ten or eleven, I noticed I had no further lower back pain. I crawled for a few more days, and continued to feel completely healed. At that point, I lessened up on the crawling, and soon stopped altogether when I realized that my cure seemed to be permanent.

I returned to my life, to the same habits, the same lifestyle, with a completely healed lower back. Best of all, I didn't need to keep crawling to maintain the healing. Of course, I was prepared to resume crawling if the pain returned, but it never did. It's been comforting to know I have this certain cure to turn to for lower back pain, if I ever needed it again.

Update: as time passed, I eventually added crawling to my morning exercise routine just to enjoy its general health benefits, and recommend you do so as well. The good news is, ten years later, I am still experiencing a completely pain-free lower back!

Chapter 4

The Science Behind The Method

Contrary to popular belief, crawling isn't just a means of transportation for infants; it is a critical developmental stage that builds a healthy brain and body. However, most people can't imagine why they should continue to crawl once they have learned to walk. The research is in, and crawling has been used, among other things, to alleviate brain disorders in children, teens and adults, support healthy childbirth, help with weight loss, increase muscle strength in army commandos, and, last but not least, treat and prevent lower back pain. Let us look at some of the scientific data.

Brain Integration

A link has been established between ADHD and the Symmetric Tonic Neck Reflex, otherwise known as the 'crawling reflex.' If an infant crawls sufficiently, they automatically release the crawling reflex, which in turn enables them to fully develop both hemispheres of their brain. However, many people who suffer from ADHD did not crawl at all or enough during their early years. Therefore, by crawling as a child, teen or adult, they can help release this reflex and ultimately reduce ADHD symptoms, which include inability to concentrate, difficulty learning and impulsive behavior.

Carla Hannaford states in her book, *Smart Moves: Why Learning Is Not All In Your Head,* that crawling in infancy is absolutely vital for coordinating the two hemispheres of the brain. She discovered that babies need to crawl around 50,000 times in order to fully establish the neuronal connections in their brain system. If they do not do so, it can hamper their ability to learn.

The repetitive nature of the crawling movement is what enables the two hemispheres of the brain to integrate, thus improving attention, concentration, memory, logical thinking and more. Dr. Lise Eliot, Associate Professor of Neuroscience at The Chicago Medical School of Rosalind Franklin University of Medicine and Science, has determined that crawling increases myelin production in the brain, allowing nerve signals to travel up to 100 times faster.

Adults can take advantage of this research, especially if they didn't crawl enough when they were infants. The latest CMRI studies reveal the plasticity of the brain and show that brain cells continue to develop and increase in number throughout life if properly stimulated. Crawling as an adult stimulates both sides of the brain and allows you to develop your brain in areas that may not have been fully developed as an infant. For adults who did crawl sufficiently as infants, it can increase the integration of the right and left sides of the brain, thereby enhancing cognitive and creative abilities, and improving mood. The point is, it is never too late to more fully develop your brain or prevent brain aging, and you can easily do so through crawling!

Weight Loss

Crawling is one of the best exercises for helping you lose weight. The reason for this is that crawling engages more muscles simultaneously than any other type of exercise. This in turn requires the expenditure of significantly more energy, resulting in your burning fat and increasing your metabolic rate. A 2010 research study, reported in the "Journal of Comparative Physiology," evaluated quadruped (four-legged) animals and their fat burning process during exercise. From these animal studies, the authors concluded that crawling is likely to help people lose weight, especially from the stomach, butt and thighs, with additional research indicating that it also helps shed arm fat.

The American Council on Exercise further states that there are numerous ways in which the human body benefits from crawling. This includes losing weight and building up muscle strength for other activities.

I hope you are beginning to see how crawling not only helps you lose weight, but it is also one of the best ways to make sure all of the muscles in your body are getting a good work out.

Preventing Breech Birth

Books such as *Birthways: Natural Measures for Turning a Breech Baby* have shown that crawling greatly benefits women who are about to give birth. This is because it helps rotate the fetus in the womb, which means that the fetus moves into the correct head first position for birth. Adding a bit of crawling to your exercise program during pregnancy will virtually eradicate the chance of your having a breech birth. However, be sure to check with your doctor first.

Diagnosing Autism

Crawling is used to diagnose autism in infants; their movements can be analyzed long before they can speak. This enables parents to cope with their child's autism at a much earlier stage and initiate the appropriate treatment.

Back Health

Throughout your day to day life, gravity has a constant effect on your body. This is evidenced by the fact that you actually shrink during the day by around 1/2 an inch. During the evening, moisture returns to your spinal discs, which allows you to 'grow' again. Over time, however, your body will tend to succumb to the effects of gravity, and this in turn can lead to spinal problems. A horizontal exercise regime is normally prescribed by doctors for those who are suffering from back pain.

Crawling is an excellent horizontal exercise because it removes pressure from the spine, which means you are less likely to suffer from slipped discs and curvature of the spine over time. In fact, crawling helps retain the original curvature of the spine you had as a baby. This realignment of your spine virtually eliminates any back pain you may have due to the effects of gravity. Studies have shown that four-legged animals never experience back pain or back disorders due to the reduced pressure of gravity on their musculo-skeletal structure. Isn't it obvious how crawling exercises can be beneficial for your lower back?

Army Training

The army still regularly teaches crawling during basic training. The reason for this is because it develops the muscle strength and agility that allows soldiers to stay low while covering large amounts of distance quickly.

FitCrawl

For crawling aficionados, a company named 'FitCrawl' has designed a machine to help capitalize on all the benefits mentioned above. Their exercise machine enables you to practice your crawling movements in place, without having to crawl on the floor in an open space. Check it out at www.fitcrawl.com.

As you can see, crawling is vital to the development of a child. Many learning and mental health issues that older kids, teens and adults experience are related to not crawling sufficiently or properly as an infant. The good news is that most of these issues can be eliminated at any age by following a regular crawling program. The additional health benefits of crawling, such as weight loss, increased muscle strength and back health, make this exercise too important to pass up. If you are an adult and have yet to engage in crawling as an exercise, then I strongly suggest you do. It will do your body a world of good, as well as possibly eliminate many of the problems that have been plaguing you throughout your life.

Sources:

http://www.centeredge.com/ArticPDF/STNR.pdf

http://www.hoofbeats.us/

http://www.fitcrawl.com.au

http://www.acefitness.org/exerciselibrary/150/bear-crawl

http://usmilitary.about.com/od/airforcejoin/a/afbmtbeast.htm

Chapter 5

The Ten Essentials

If you decide to take up crawling, read this chapter before you begin. It contains an important checklist of things you need to consider.

1. Crawl every day for two weeks to give this technique a chance to heal your lower back pain. The effects on your spine are cumulative and the results are faster and more certain if you do a little bit every day.

2. Do use a timer and start at no more than 30 seconds. Expect to take ten days or more to build up to crawling for five minutes per session.

Remember, a little goes a long way, and you never need crawl for more than a few minutes to achieve tremendous benefits. The idea is not to strain yourself in any way. Just work within your comfort level during each session.

3. Try it first without the knee pads. You may not need them as not everyone has sensitive knees. Plus, you can always purchase them down the road. If, however, you know your knees are vulnerable, do make sure to have them on hand from the start. Our recommended brand is listed in the resources section of this book.

4. You don't need any special clothing; just make sure your clothes are loose enough to move with ease, but not so loose that they get in your way.

5. You may want to crawl in private, as some people feel embarrassed being observed by family members on all fours doing the crawling exercise.

6. Always make sure to allow your head to fall in the natural downward position when crawling, as crawling with your head lifted up

can cause neck strain. You can gently bend your head to the right or left when crawling to help you see where you're going.

7. Choose a clear path ahead of time, like a long hallway, so you don't feel the need to look up and ahead to make sure you won't run into anything. But if ever uncertain, just gently bend your head to the right or left to help you see where you're going.

8. As you become more comfortable with crawling, experiment with different crawling techniques or try varying the speed of your crawling. View it as a playful exercise and change up your techniques whenever you get bored or need a bigger challenge. In the resource section of this book, there are links to websites that demonstrate additional crawling techniques to add to your armament, including the bear crawl.

9. If you have any concerns at all about getting up off the floor, do not try crawling unless someone is there who can help you get up if necessary. Begin your crawling regimen by

practicing getting up by yourself. One way to get up off the floor, if you are having difficulty doing so, is to crawl over to a sturdy couch or chair and pull yourself up onto it. Just make sure to try this under safe conditions, meaning with someone else present. In the resources section of this book, there is a link to a website with instructions for seniors, as well as a link to a video demonstrating how to get up off the floor.

10. If you have health conditions that affect your knees, shoulders, neck or back, or any other health concerns, check with your doctor first to make sure that crawling is a good exercise for you.

Chapter 6

Using Your Intuition to Heal Your Body

When I healed my lower back pain by following my intuition, no one could have been more surprised than me that it worked! I had been experiencing vague mental images and an urge to hit the ground crawling for months before I finally decided to give in to it.

At first, the inner voice, which is what I call the part of me that was presenting these images and urges, was faint. It's not as if it arrived full-blown: "Here, do this." No, not at all. It came as vague images, vague ideas and vague sensations, so distant and seemingly remote they were easy to ignore, that is, until I reached my endpoint after a year of suffering with no respite. During that entire time, my lower back pain had limited my enjoyment of everyday life and threatened to ruin a long-planned and otherwise amazing trip abroad.

I encourage you to tune into and pay attention to any inner guidance you may be getting about your lower back pain. Though abundantly backed by scientific research, my solution may not be *your* solution since no solution fits everyone; and what I really want is for you to find *your* solution, the one that ends your lower back pain.

Having said that, I certainly hope that you give my method a full two week try before going in a new direction. Our culture does not make it easy to trust yourself to find your own cures by listening to your inner voice, and my method could quickly bring an end to your problem like it has for so many of my readers. But if for some reason it does not, the next step is to learn how to focus within to identify any messages you may be receiving from your inner self. Here are some techniques that I have used successfully to resolve health and other issues.

Talk to Your Body

I have found that talking to the part of your body that hurts, and 'listening' for a response can be a fast track solution for solving body issues. Here's how it works. Begin by viewing the hurting part of you as a beloved pet or a small child, both of whom know on some level that their survival depends upon you. Ask it whether there is something it would like to tell you about why it's hurting.

By listening for a response, I literally mean listening, in the sense that the response will come as images or words in your mind, or both. Don't be afraid of your own mind! It's a powerful healing tool and can give you all the answers you need, if only you would trust it.

As an example, your body might tell you, "I feel afraid." You would then say, "What are you afraid of?" That conversation might go like this:

Body: That you will not take care of me.

You: Why do you feel that way?

Body: Because you pay very little attention to me and I feel neglected.

You: What are you afraid will happen if I don't take better care of you?

Body: I will be so neglected I might die!

You: Oh, I am so sorry for not paying more attention to you! Please know you are safe, and I will keep you safe. What do you need me to do?

Body: I need exercise, fresh air and sunlight every day.

You: You got it. I will do that for you from now on. If I do that, will you stop hurting?

Body: Yes, except I want my muscles to be stretched every day too - do some spine rolls, toe touches or crawling before we go out.

You: Of course, little one, I will. Will that make you feel loved and cared for?

Body: Yes.

You: Will that make my lower back stop hurting?

Body: Yes, if you do that every day for two weeks. Then you have to keep it up or I will hurt again.

You: You got it, little one, I will do that every day and we will be happy together.

Meditate

Having a conversation with your body is one way of learning what your body needs from you in order for it to be free of lower back pain. Another method is to meditate every day by sitting quietly for at least 10 minutes, and allowing yourself to float like a cork on water – no goal, no effort, no thought. Whatever thoughts do come up, let them pass through without pondering them. After 10 minutes or when you feel very quiet inside, ask your lower back, 'What can I do to heal you?' Or, 'What do you need in order to heal?' And then, listen for the answer, which will likely come as words and/or images in your mind.

These techniques can be used to help you get to the bottom of your lower back pain. I have found that, while stress – meaning negative emotions like fear, frustration, anger and grief – may be a factor in causing pain, there are often environmental components as well. These may include something you are doing that is causing the pain, such as lifting heavy items or lifting from a wrong position, or something you are not doing. The latter may include a simple lack of self-care like not drinking enough water, not getting up from a seated position on a regular basis, not getting out and moving around, or not performing an exercise that will stretch out the lower back and realign the spine.

Usually the solution is a simple one like crawling was for me. And yes, I also do observe a schedule around how long I allow myself to sit before getting up and moving about. I also do walk outdoors every day, get a little sunshine and fresh air, and stay hydrated. This, plus some early day stretching and bending, and a bit of time on my recumbent bike, keep me limber and pain free all these years.

The point is – you can't indulge in being a couch potato if you want to sustain the benefits of a lower back pain cure. And you can't keep ignoring the signals when you lift something the wrong way or something that's too heavy, or you use a desk chair at work that does not provide enough lumbar support. If you persist in ignoring these triggers, you may not be able to sustain your gains.

And, finally, maintaining basic, healthy, everyday life habits goes a long way to keeping you fit as a fiddle well into your older years. Ask yourself, would you deprive your pets or plants of fresh air, sunshine, outdoor exercise, water and healthy food? Certainly not! Now is the time to acknowledge that you deserve and have as much need for these things as they do.

Whatever method you use to rid yourself of lower back pain – whether it's my simple crawling technique or something you discover that works for you – continue to use it. By combining the right exercise with healthy daily habits, I can virtually guarantee you will heal and sustain your healing.

You probably realize by now that my personal bias is to avoid the medical scenario whenever possible. I do this because I believe the body is capable of healing itself if given the right natural support. I also like feeling in charge of my own body and enjoy finding natural solutions to health issues. In my experience, many ailments can be prevented or cured with the kind of attention to and care of the body that I describe in this chapter.

If you are considering a medical solution, why not first try the crawling and lifestyle changes suggested here, and/or take the time to tune into your own inner voice and see where that leads you. I feel confident you will be as amazed as I was when I followed my inner voice and cured my year long, chronic lower back pain in ten days, with only a few minutes a day of crawling!

Disclaimer

Dear reader, since I don't know you or the cause of your lower back pain, nor am I a medical doctor, please do not misconstrue the above as medical advice. Sometimes, the fastest and easiest solution is medical. Sometimes, an ailment clearly requires medical intervention or a person needs to feel supported by a medical professional in order to heal. Therefore, I encourage you to consult your doctor before trying my method.

Conclusion

The Best Natural Strategies

More people than ever before suffer from lower back pain because of our sedentary culture. However, the good news is, the same techniques that help you overcome lower back problems will also help you prevent them. Here is a summary of the four best natural strategies for maintaining a healthy lower back.

Lose Weight

If you are overweight, the first thing you should do is lose weight. For many people, carrying around excess weight can make a difference in your overall lower back health. This is because the spine tends to buckle and even compress beneath the additional weight. To compensate for the extra weight, your hips may also shift forward and pinch your sciatic nerve. Just by losing weight, you may find that your lower back pain eases or goes away.

Exercise

The second thing you must do is get regular exercise. A thirty minute daily walk is an excellent overall body tonic. Working your core muscles with a series of gentle movements, such as Tai Chi, Pilates or yoga, can do a lot to help you strengthen your lower back. Simple stretching in the morning, even before you get out of bed, can also be an excellent way to prevent lower back pain. If you keep this area of your body limber, lower back problems are less likely to occur.

Drink Water

Third, make sure that you are hydrated properly. Drinking 8 or more glasses of water every day, along with taking some natural sea salt, will ensure that you are not experiencing lower back pain as a result of dehydration. Not only can it help with your lower back, but it can also help with your overall health, and the results are rather quick to occur.

Crawl

And, finally, try the ultimate lower back pain cure – crawling. Whether you crawl to heal yourself of lower back pain as I did, or crawl as the perfect preventative, the main thing is, do it! All I can say is, it works, folks, it works beyond your wildest dreams!

Integrating these practices with your daily life is the best way to overcome lower back pain and keep it from reoccurring. The effort you put into taking care of your lower back is going to pay off big by an absence of pain in your life.

You can succeed in being free of lower back pain if you follow the guidelines in this book. Just make sure to consult with your doctor first, then take action on what you have learned. I am confident crawling will help you like it helped me!

Before you go, please don't forget to contact us for your bonus gift, *Lower Back Pain Free!: Discover The 10 Best Ways to Cure Lower Back Pain Naturally*. The information in that ebook perfectly complements the main method I teach in *When Nothing Else Works*. It reveals additional natural and easy ways to help heal and prevent lower back pain. Together, these two books provide everything you need to know to keep your lower back happy and healthy.

To receive your free gift all you have to do is send an email to info@diamondstarpress.com along with proof of purchase and "Send Lower Back Pain Gift" in the subject field, and we will get your bonus out to you right away. Do it now before you forget!

Resources

Here are some recommended websites and products to assist you in becoming lower back pain free.

Websites

http://lmb.typepad.com/smart_senior/2009/10/senior-exercise-getting-up-off-from-the-floor.html/ - Instructions on how to get on and off the floor for seniors.

http://www.youtube.com/watch?v=HB6WMasb3vM/ – A helpful YouTube video on how to get off the floor using the "reach and roll" method.

http://www.thatsfit.com/2009/10/09/bear-crawl-for-tight-abs/ - This an excellent video on how to do the bear crawl forward and back-ward.

http://physicalliving.com/how-to-move-on-all-fours/ - Instructions and video on a variety of crawling techniques.

http://en.wikipedia.org/wiki/Crawling_(human)/ - Information on different types of crawling exercises.

Products

Knee Pads – I use and highly recommend Work-Force brand Durable Foam Knee Pads, Model No. 171-300, for crawling exercises. This is a strong, yet lightweight knee pad with Velcro straps. It costs approximately $8.99 and can be purchased, if you live in the US, at Home Depot. For other excellent knee pad options, visit Amazon.com. If you have especially sensitive knees, be sure to check out their gel knee pad options.

Did You Enjoy This Book?

Dear Reader,

Thank you for reading this book. I hope you enjoyed *When Nothing Else Works: How To Cure Your Lower Back Pain Fast!*

My purpose in writing this book is to reveal my discovery that a simple crawling exercise, performed in a specific way, was able to permanently heal my chronic lower back pain when nothing else worked. By sharing this information, my hope is that it will help you heal your lower back pain too.

If you would like to help me reach other readers with this valuable information, please write a review on Amazon now. It will only take a few minutes, and I would appreciate it very much!

Thanks again, and wishing you the best of health!

S. F. Howe

Books by S. F. Howe

MIND · BODY · SPIRIT

HIGHER CONSCIOUSNESS

Matrix Man: How To Become Enlightened, Happy And Free In An Illusion World

The author reveals a new reality paradigm that will liberate you from the limiting beliefs and programs that prevent a joyful and fulfilling life. Available in print and digital editions.

The Top Ten Myths Of Enlightenment: Exposing The Truth About Spiritual Enlightenment That Will Set You Free!

Essential reading for spiritual seekers. What no one else will tell you to help you avoid the pitfalls of the spiritual journey. Available in print and digital editions.

The Bringer Discourses: On Waking Up To The Mind Control Programs Of The Matrix Reality

For those seeking freedom from cultural indoctrination, this book offers a higher dimensional perspective on the most ingrained and unquestioned aspects of everyday life and has the ability to heal and awaken humanity. Available in print and digital editions.

PLANT INTELLIGENCE

Secrets Of The Plant Whisperer: How To Care For, Connect, And Communicate With Your House Plants

A plant whisperer reveals the hidden truth about plants and why relating to them in a conscious way is vital for their health and well-being. Available in print and digital editions.

Your Plant Speaks!: How To Use Your Houseplant As A Therapist

Let your house plant solve your problems! Discover the little known art of receiving life coaching from your favorite indoor plant.
Coming Soon!

PERSONAL GROWTH

Vision Board Success: How To Get Everything You Want With Vision Boards!

A powerful technique for achieving your goals and manifesting your desires. Available in print and digital editions.

Sex Yoga: The 7 Easy Steps To A Mind-Blowing Kundalini Awakening!

A technique for activating the chakras to induce a powerful kundalini experience. Available in print and digital editions.

Morning Routine For Night Owls: How To Supercharge Your Day With A Gentle Yet Powerful Morning Routine!

Morning rituals aren't only for morning people, and they don't have to be rough and tumble or performed at top speed to set up a perfect day. Welcome to the world of the gentle yet powerful wake-up routine for night owls! Available in print and digital editions.

CONSCIOUS HEALTH

Transgender America: Spirit, Identity, & The Emergence Of The Third Gender

A higher consciousness perspective on the Transgender Agenda; what it is and why it is being rolled out at breakneck speed to social engineer a gender dysphoria epidemic. Available in print and digital editions.

When Nothing Else Works: How To Cure Your Lower Back Pain Fast!

The simple method that no doctor will ever tell you about. Requires no drugs, no surgery, and no special equipment. Available in print and digital editions.

About the Author

S. F. Howe is a psychologist, author and spiritual teacher. Howe received a master's degree and doctoral training in clinical psychology, and worked in hospitals and clinics for more than 25 years as a psychotherapist, staff psychologist, clinical program consultant and director of chemical dependency and psychiatric programs.

In the midst of graduate studies, a profound spiritual awakening led to a complete reevaluation of the author's life path. Thus began a spiritual journey along the road less traveled, extending far beyond clinical psychology, conventional reality paradigms and both traditional religion and new age spirituality.

While engaged in a unique, ongoing process of discovery, the author enjoys sharing with others an ever-expanding understanding of the true nature of personal reality. This has resulted in Howe's noted books and teachings on the subjects of higher consciousness, conscious health, plant intelligence and personal growth. Howe's primary intention is to bring an end to suffering by guiding others on a well-worn path to truth and expanded awareness. Many of those who have experienced Howe's input and presence report emotional and physical healing, life-changing realizations and dramatic personal transformation.

S. F. Howe may be contacted for speaking and teaching engagements. Please direct all inquiries to info@diamondstarpress.com.

Made in the USA
Middletown, DE
08 August 2021

45655251R00040